The Patient's Guide to Mitochondrial Dysfunction

Diagnosis, Treatment and Hope

Travis Jenkins

Table of Contents

Introduction

The complicated illness known as mitochondrial dysfunction can take many different forms. Individualized treatment strategies and a multidisciplinary approach are necessary for the disease's diagnosis and management. For patients and their families, The Patient's Guide to Mitochondrial Dysfunction offers thorough information about the illness, including diagnosis, treatment options, and hope. Guidelines for screening, referrals to specialists, and drugs that should be used cautiously in individuals with mitochondria are all included in the handbook. It also emphasizes how crucial it is to have an emergency care plan on hand that describes the underlying condition in depth and offers management guidelines. Based on a global consensus of knowledgeable experts in mitochondrial disease, the guide is meant to supplement the 2015 consensus statement "Diagnosis and Management of Mitochondrial Disease."

- Understanding Mitochondrial Dysfunction

Small organelles in cells called mitochondria are responsible for energy production. A class of hereditary disorders known as mitochondrial illnesses, which impact how mitochondria generate energy within the body, can be brought on by dysfunctional mitochondria. Numerous body parts, including the brain, muscles, and organs, might be affected by the diverse range of symptoms associated with mitochondrial illness. Muscle biopsies, DNA testing, and blood and urine tests can all be used to diagnose mitochondrial illness. There is currently no known cure; however, treatment can help manage symptoms and delay the course of the illness. Individuals who have mitochondrial disease ought to have an emergency care plan with them that describes their underlying condition and offers guidelines for treatment. Standardized care and preventive medical attention should be provided to patients with primary mitochondrial illnesses. For patients with mitochondrial disease, genetic counseling for couples, family history analysis, and prenatal diagnosis are crucial. Individuals who have mitochondrial disease should stay away from circumstances that could exacerbate their symptoms because they are more vulnerable right after becoming ill.

- Importance of Patient Empowerment

The Patient's Guide to Mitochondrial Dysfunction: Diagnosis, Treatment, and Hope highlights the significance of patient empowerment.

A vital component of healthcare is patient empowerment, particularly in the intricate area of mitochondrial medicine. Giving patients the information, abilities, and tools they need to properly manage their health and wellbeing is a key component of patient empowerment. Better results, a higher standard of living, and more efficient use of healthcare resources are all possible with this strategy. When it comes to mitochondrial dysfunction, patient empowerment is crucial for comprehending the illness, navigating the diagnostic procedure, and selecting the best course of action.

Advantages of Patient Involvement

1. Better patient outcomes: Patients who feel empowered are more likely to take charge of their

care, follow through on treatment plans, and comprehend their condition.

2. Improved quality of life: Patients who are able to take charge of their own health have a higher standard of living since they are more equipped to make decisions regarding their care and way of living.

3. More efficient use of healthcare resources: Patients who feel empowered are more likely to make appropriate use of healthcare resources, which lowers the need for needless hospital stays and ER visits.

4. Better coping strategies: Patients who are given the tools to take charge of their health can learn useful coping mechanisms to handle symptoms like exhaustion, discomfort, and energy loss that come with having a mitochondrial disease.

Techniques for Giving Patients Power

1. Education: Give patients current, accurate information about their disease, available treatments, and lifestyle choices that will enable them to properly manage their health.

2. Communication: Promote candid and open dialogue among patients, their medical professionals, and their support system to

guarantee that everyone is aware of the patient's condition and on the same page.

3. Involvement in decision-making: Give patients the opportunity to actively participate in treatment planning and decision-making by involving them in the decision-making processes linked to their care.

4. Access to resources: Assist patients in taking better care of their conditions and making educated decisions about their treatment by providing them with pertinent resources, including professional services, educational materials, and support groups.

5. Regular monitoring and follow-up: To monitor the patient's development, evaluate their reaction to therapy, and make any required modifications to their care plan, set up a regular monitoring and follow-up schedule.

As a result, patient empowerment plays a critical role in the patient's guide to mitochondrial dysfunction. By empowering patients to take charge of their health, quality of life and health outcomes are all improved, and healthcare resources are used more efficiently. Healthcare professionals can empower patients to take an active role in their care by arming them with the information, abilities, and tools they need, which will eventually enhance their general health.

Chapter One

Demystifying Mitochondrial Dysfunction

When the mitochondria, the parts of cells that produce energy, are not able to operate correctly, it is known as mitochondrial dysfunction. This may result in a class of hereditary disorders called mitochondrial illnesses, which impact the body's ability to produce energy. Mitochondrial illnesses can affect the brain, muscles, and organs, among other aspects of the body. They can also result in serious symptoms and problems. While there isn't a cure for mitochondrial illnesses at this time, there are treatments that can help control symptoms and stop potentially fatal consequences. Together with their medical professionals, patients with mitochondrial disorders should create a thorough care plan that takes into account all of their unique requirements and difficulties. Furthermore, in order to enable people with mitochondrial disorders to better understand their condition and take an active role in their care, patient education and empowerment are essential. This will eventually improve the quality of life and health outcomes for those affected.

1.1 What Are Mitochondria and Their Role?

What Is the Function of Mitochondria? The Patient's Handbook of Mitochondrial Dysfunction: Identification, Management, and Prospects

Almost all of the body's cells include tiny, energy-producing organelles called mitochondria. They are important for the production of ATP, which is needed for the correct operation of cells and organs. Particularly crucial are mitochondria in organs with high energy requirements, like the heart, muscles, and brain. When the mitochondria cannot operate correctly, it results in mitochondrial dysfunction, which is the cause of a class of hereditary disorders known as mitochondrial illnesses. These illnesses can produce severe symptoms and consequences and can affect practically any region of the body, including the brain, muscles, and organs.

Mutations in either the nuclear DNA (nDNA) or the mitochondrial DNA (mtDNA) can result in mitochondrial disorders. Depending on the particular illness type and the organs impacted, the symptoms of mitochondrial diseases might differ greatly. Muscle weakness, exhaustion, difficulties with hearing and vision, digestive disorders, and developmental delays are typical symptoms.

Muscle biopsies, DNA testing, and blood and urine tests can all be used to diagnose mitochondrial disorders. There is presently no recognized cure for mitochondrial illnesses; however, treatment can help manage symptoms and decrease the disease's course. Medication, vitamins, physical therapy, and lifestyle changes are all possible forms of treatment.

To sum up, mitochondria are vital components of cells that are critical to the process of energy production. A class of hereditary disorders known as mitochondrial illnesses, which can affect practically every region of the body and result in severe symptoms and problems, can be attributed to mitochondrial dysfunction. Patients should collaborate closely with their healthcare professionals to create a comprehensive care plan that covers their unique requirements and problems, as the diagnosis and treatment of mitochondrial illnesses can be complicated.

1.2 Common Causes of Mitochondrial Dysfunction

The Patient's Guide to Mitochondrial Dysfunction: Diagnosis, Treatment, and Hope lists the following common causes of mitochondrial dysfunction:.

Numerous things, including lifestyle choices, environmental pollutants, and genetic abnormalities, can lead to mitochondrial malfunction. Mutations in either the nuclear DNA (nDNA) or the mitochondrial DNA (mtDNA) are usually the cause of mitochondrial disorders. Numerous symptoms and consequences may result from these abnormalities that impact the mitochondria's ability to operate.

The following are a few typical reasons for mitochondrial dysfunction:

1. Genetic mutations: Alterations in the mtDNA or nDNA might cause mitochondrial disorders by compromising the mitochondria's ability to function.

2. Environmental poisons: Exposure to chemicals, heavy metals, and pesticides, among other environmental toxins, can harm and disrupt the mitochondria's function.

3. Lifestyle factors: Chronic stress, poor diet, and inactivity can all lead to mitochondrial dysfunction.

4. Pharmaceuticals: Antibiotics and chemotherapy treatments are two examples of pharmaceuticals that might harm mitochondria and disrupt their function.

5. Age: As people age, their mitochondrial function normally decreases, which may play a role in the emergence of mitochondrial diseases.

Muscle biopsies, DNA testing, and blood and urine tests can all be used to diagnose mitochondrial disorders. There is presently no recognized cure for mitochondrial illnesses; however, treatment can help manage symptoms and decrease the disease's course. Medication, vitamins, physical therapy, and lifestyle changes are all possible forms of treatment.

In conclusion, a range of factors, including genetic abnormalities, environmental pollutants, and lifestyle choices, can lead to mitochondrial malfunction. Together with their medical professionals, patients with mitochondrial disorders should create a thorough care plan that takes into account all of their unique requirements and difficulties. Furthermore, in order to enable people with mitochondrial disorders to better understand their condition and take an active role in their care, patient education and empowerment are essential. This will eventually improve the quality of life and health outcomes for those affected.

Chapter Two

Recognizing Symptoms and Seeking Diagnosis

A class of illnesses known as mitochondrial diseases damage the mitochondria, which are microscopic organelles found in every cell in the body and are in charge of generating energy. Mitochondrial disease symptoms can develop at any age, but they can also be evident from birth. They can be minor to severe and include changes in vision, hearing, and organ function, as well as muscle weariness, weakness, and sensitivity to certain types of exercise. Even among members of the same family, there are significant differences in the intensity of each of these symptoms. In the event that you are experiencing severe symptoms, such as breathing difficulties or a seizure, dial 911 or your local emergency services number right away. A medical professional typically notices symptoms that impact many organs or organ systems simultaneously. Speak with a physician or genetic counselor if you think you or a loved one may have a mitochondrial disease. While there is no known treatment for mitochondrial illnesses, it is possible to manage symptoms. Your care team will be there to support you as you navigate this diagnosis and your treatment options, in addition to the assistance of your family and friends.

2.1 Identifying Early Warning Signs

A wide range of symptoms can be present with mitochondrial abnormalities, and it can be challenging to recognize early warning indications. On the other hand, low muscle tone, weariness, gastrointestinal issues, developmental delay, and intolerance to exercise are some common symptoms. Additional symptoms could be vomiting, severe constipation, nausea, seizures, blindness, cardiomyopathy, deafness, dementia, feeding issues, frequent infections, irregular heartbeat, increased fatigue, migraine headaches, muscle weakness, nausea, and symptoms similar to a stroke. Speak with a healthcare professional if you or a loved one is exhibiting any of these signs. To help establish whether a mitochondrial problem is present, a physical examination, blood tests, particular mitochondrial and/or nuclear gene testing, brain magnetic resonance imaging (MRI), EKG, echocardiography, eye exam, neurological evaluation, and hearing test may be utilized. In the event that a mitochondrial issue is identified, therapy can help control symptoms and enhance life expectancy.

2.2 Diagnostic Tests and Procedures

For the purpose of diagnosing mitochondrial disease, a thorough approach is taken to evaluate mitochondrial function and pinpoint related symptoms. These could consist of:

1. Blood Tests: Genetic testing, blood enzyme tests, and plasma lactate levels are frequently employed. Long-standing evidence of mitochondrial illness has been linked to elevated lactate levels, yet this result is not diagnostically necessary. Tests for blood enzymes, like serum creatine kinase, can reveal an electron transport chain deficit.

2. Biopsy Testing: Mitochondrial alterations can be directly detected by muscle or other tissue biopsies. In particular, a muscle biopsy can be very helpful in diagnosing diseases of the muscles. It is crucial to remember that the absence of mitochondrial alterations in a biopsy from one type of tissue does not rule out the possibility that the same changes exist in other body sections.

3. Imaging: Structural abnormalities can be detected by brain magnetic resonance imaging (MRI) and other imaging modalities.

4. Functional Tests: Tests of strength and endurance, such as an exercise test, can be used to evaluate mitochondrial function, as can polarographic analysis to quantify integrated mitochondrial oxidative phosphorylation (OXPHOS) capacity.

5. Genetic Testing: To determine the underlying molecular etiology causing primary mitochondrial illness, molecular testing is necessary. This is now regarded as a typical step in the diagnostic procedure and is crucial for verifying the diagnosis.

It is crucial to stress that a combination of these tests and the knowledge of medical professionals is frequently used in the diagnosis of mitochondrial illness. The field of mitochondrial medicine is always changing, and methods for testing and developing diagnostic criteria are updated and improved upon frequently.

2.3 Importance of Timely Diagnosis

For mitochondrial illness to be effectively managed and treated, a prompt diagnosis is essential. Diagnosing mitochondrial illnesses can be difficult due to their complexity and heterogeneity in presentation. Nonetheless, prompt diagnosis can enhance patients' quality of life by halting more bodily harm. A "diagnostic odyssey," which can last for several years and result in severe stress and anguish for patients and their families, can be brought on by a delayed diagnosis. Consequently, when assessing patients exhibiting symptoms that could be linked to mitochondrial dysfunction, primary care doctors should be knowledgeable about mitochondrial illnesses and take them into account when making a differential diagnosis. To confirm a diagnosis of mitochondrial illness, a complete diagnostic strategy may be required, involving blood tests, biopsy testing, imaging, functional tests, and genetic testing. Appropriate treatment can be started as soon as a diagnosis is made to control symptoms and enhance quality of life. In conclusion, prompt diagnosis of mitochondrial disease is critical to the best possible care and therapy of the illness.

Chapter 3

Navigating the Medical Landscape

Because mitochondrial dysfunction is a complex disorder with few well-defined diagnostic criteria, patients may find it difficult to navigate the medical system. Nonetheless, patients and their medical professionals can more successfully manage the condition if they are aware of the main features of mitochondrial diseases and the available treatment choices. The following are some crucial things to think about:

1. "Complexity of Mitochondrial Diseases": A diverse range of illnesses with differing clinical manifestations and degrees of severity include mitochondrial diseases. Healthcare practitioners find it challenging to detect and treat many illnesses due to their complexity.

2. Diagnostic Challenges: The absence of sensitive and particular biomarkers makes diagnosing mitochondrial illnesses difficult. Furthermore, since the field of mitochondrial medicine is developing quickly, additional information may need to be included in the diagnostic criteria.

3. Integrated Approach: For the proper clinical management of mitochondrial illnesses, an integrated approach to diagnosis that incorporates clinical, histological, biochemical, and genetic assessment is necessary.

4. Treatment Options: A number of treatments are available to manage symptoms and enhance quality of life, despite the fact that there is no known cure for mitochondrial illnesses. Exercise, hearing aids, and lowering toxic metabolites are a few possible therapy options.

5. Clinical Trials: New methods for diagnosis and therapy are being investigated in the field of mitochondrial medicine, which is a sector that is always changing. Enrolling in these trials can help patients and their families gain access to new treatments and progress in the field of mitochondrial medicine.

6. Support and Education: Groups like the Mitochondrial Medicine Society and the United Mitochondrial Disease Foundation (UMDF) provide information and support to patients and their families. These groups support more awareness and funding for research while also

connecting sufferers with doctors and offering services.

In summary, people with mitochondrial dysfunction must navigate the medical system with a thorough grasp of the illness, the difficulties associated with diagnosis, and the range of possible treatments. Patients can have access to the best available diagnostic and therapeutic methods by staying up-to-date on the most recent developments in mitochondrial medicine and by taking part in clinical studies.

3.1 Building a Supportive Healthcare Team

Establishing a healthcare team that is supportive is crucial for individuals suffering from mitochondrial dysfunction. Healthcare professionals have a difficult time diagnosing and treating mitochondrial diseases due to the condition's complexity and the absence of clear diagnostic guidelines. Consequently, it is critical that patients have access to a team of medical specialists who can offer complete care and are educated in mitochondrial disorders. The following people are essential components of a caring medical team:

1. Primary Care Physician: For patients with mitochondrial dysfunction, a primary care physician is frequently the initial point of contact. They can assist in monitoring general health, referring patients to experts, and coordinating care.

2. Mitochondrial Disease Specialist: A doctor with experience in identifying and managing mitochondrial disorders is known as a mitochondrial disease specialist. They can offer customized care and solutions for treatment based on the individual needs of the patient.

3. Genetic Counselor: An expert in mitochondrial disorders and their effects on future generations, a genetic counselor can assist patients and their families in comprehending the genetic foundation of these conditions. They can also offer advice on family planning and genetic testing.

4. Physical Therapist: Patients with mitochondrial dysfunction can enhance their strength, stamina, and range of motion with the assistance of a physical therapist. They can also offer advice on changing activities and getting exercise.

5. Occupational Therapist: An occupational therapist can assist individuals suffering from

mitochondrial dysfunction in enhancing their capacity to carry out daily tasks, including getting dressed, taking care of themselves, and cooking.

6. Nutritionist: A nutritionist can assist individuals with mitochondrial dysfunction in creating a diet that is both healthy and tailored to their individual dietary requirements.

7. Social Worker: A social worker can assist patients and their families in navigating the healthcare system, finding resources, and dealing with the financial strain of their illness. They can also offer emotional support.

In conclusion, creating a healthcare team that is supportive is crucial for individuals who suffer from mitochondrial dysfunction. Patients can improve their quality of life and effectively manage their condition with the assistance of a team of healthcare professionals who are knowledgeable about mitochondrial diseases and can provide comprehensive care.

3.2 Communicating Effectively with Healthcare Professionals

Patients with mitochondrial dysfunction must communicate effectively with healthcare providers. A patient's care can be greatly impacted by transparent and honest communication, especially in light of the condition's complexity and the difficulties in diagnosis and treatment. The following are important things to remember when speaking with medical professionals:

1. Seeking Specialized Care: It's critical to get medical attention from specialists who specialize in mitochondrial disorders. Physicians with a concentration on mitochondrial medicine and regular scholarly involvement in the field, as well as those who are a part of the Mitochondrial Care Network (MCN), may fall under this category.

2. Providing Detailed Medical History: To assist medical specialists in comprehending the nature of the ailment and its possible genetic ramifications, furnish a thorough medical history, encompassing any familial history of mitochondrial diseases.

3. Talking About Symptoms and Issues: Express all symptoms and worries in detail, even if they don't appear connected. A thorough grasp of the patient's

history is crucial for an appropriate diagnosis and course of treatment of mitochondrial illnesses, which can manifest with a wide range of symptoms.

4. Asking About Red Flags: Find out about particular "red flag" symptoms, including hearing loss and diabetes, that can point to a possible mitochondrial issue. Comprehending these pivotal markers can aid in directing the diagnostic procedure.

5. Understanding the Diagnostic Process: It's critical to comprehend the diagnostic tests and treatments that may be suggested, especially in light of the difficulties associated with diagnosing mitochondrial illnesses. In addition to ensuring that the required actions are being performed to arrive at an accurate diagnosis, this can help control expectations.

6. Participating in Care Decisions: Take an active role in treatment planning and decision-making regarding your care. This could entail talking about prospective clinical trials, available treatment alternatives, and general disease management.

Patients with mitochondrial dysfunction can help create a more complete and individualized approach to their care by communicating effectively with healthcare experts, which will eventually enhance their quality of life and outcomes.

3.3 Advocating for Your Health

When coping with mitochondrial dysfunction, speaking out for your health is critical in order to guarantee that you get the best possible support and care. When speaking up for your health, follow these important steps:

1. Understand Your Condition: Learn about the signs and symptoms of mitochondrial illnesses as well as the many treatments that are available. With this information, you'll be able to interact with your healthcare team more successfully and make well-informed decisions regarding your care.

2. Develop a Patient Treatment Plan: Collaborate with your medical team to draft a thorough plan of treatment that takes into account your unique requirements and objectives. This strategy ought to have a thorough treatment schedule, monitoring techniques, and symptom management techniques.

3. Look for Specialized Care: Locate medical specialists who specialize in mitochondrial

illnesses, such as those connected to the United Mitochondrial Disease Foundation (UMDF) or the Mitochondrial Care Network (MCN).

4. Effective Communication: Share your symptoms, worries, and any changes in your health with your medical team in an honest and transparent manner. For an accurate diagnosis and suitable treatment to be implemented, effective communication is necessary.

5. Participate in Clinical Trials: To obtain new treatments and push the field of mitochondrial medicine forward, think about taking part in clinical trials. Clinical trials can give participants access to expert medical care and assistance.

6. Connect with Support Groups and Organizations: Join groups and organizations to meet other patients, exchange experiences, and get access to helpful resources and information. Examples of these groups and organizations include MitoAction and the UMDF.

7. Act as Your Own Advocate: If you believe that your needs are not being addressed, don't be afraid to get a second opinion or look for further resources. When it comes to overseeing your

therapy and making decisions about it, take the initiative.

You may effectively ensure that you receive the best care and support possible for your mitochondrial malfunction by speaking out for your health.

Chapter 4

Treatment Approaches and Therapeutic Options

Treatment and diagnosis of mitochondrial illnesses are difficult due to their complexity. Nonetheless, a range of therapeutic modalities and treatment techniques are available to help individuals control their symptoms and enhance their quality of life. These methods can be broadly divided into two groups: "precision medicine" methods and "one-size-fits-all" solutions.

Symptomatic therapies, primarily nutrition, exercise, exposure to hypoxia, and medication therapy, are examples of one-size-fits-all tactics. These tactics seek to boost nitric oxide synthase activity, boost mitochondrial biogenesis, boost ATP production, and enhance mitochondrial function.

The goal of precision medicine approaches is to treat a particular mitochondrial disease associated with a particular mutation or unusual metabolic signature. Gene therapy, stem cell therapy, and tailored pharmaceutical therapy are some of these methods. While stem cell therapy includes transplanting healthy stem cells to replace damaged cells, gene therapy focuses on replacing or repairing faulty mitochondrial DNA. Using medications that target particular metabolic pathways or mitochondrial proteins is known as targeted pharmacological therapy.

Patients with mitochondrial dysfunction may also benefit from supportive therapies such as occupational therapy, speech therapy, and physical therapy in addition to these treatment modalities. These treatments can enhance quality of life and aid in symptom management.

It is significant to remember that there is currently no known cure for mitochondrial illnesses and that symptom management and quality of life enhancement are the main goals of treatment. Ongoing investigations and clinical trials, however, are looking into novel therapy modalities and treatment strategies, giving patients and their families hope.

In conclusion, there are many different and developing therapy alternatives and treatment modalities for mitochondrial illnesses. A comprehensive strategy of care that incorporates supportive therapies along with precision medicine and one-size-fits-all techniques can be beneficial for patients with mitochondrial dysfunction. Patients can get the best treatment options and enhance their quality of life by collaborating closely with their healthcare team.

4.1 Medications for Mitochondrial Dysfunction

Chronic, complicated illnesses that can impact different organ systems are known as mitochondrial disorders. Although there isn't a cure for many illnesses, treatment tries to lessen symptoms and delay the course of the illness. The efficacy of available treatments varies, and continuing research aims to improve diagnostic techniques and explore possible remedies. Individuals suffering from mitochondrial illness could benefit from extra assistance and care coordination, as well as support from a multidisciplinary care team. Individuals with mitochondrial illnesses may have a wide range of prognoses, depending on a number of different circumstances.

Treatment options for mitochondrial illness could be as follows:

Dietary supplements and vitamins: These can lessen disease symptoms and delay its advancement.

Avoiding Life-Threatening Complications: The goal of treatment is to avoid potentially fatal complications.

Care Coordination: Because the disease is complex and persistent, patients may benefit from extra assistance and care coordination.

It's crucial to remember that each person will respond differently to these medicines, so before beginning any treatment, patients should talk with their healthcare professional about any possible side effects. The knowledge and management of mitochondrial illnesses are being advanced by ongoing research.

The "Mitochondrial Disease" resource from the United Mitochondrial Disease Foundation and the "Patient's Guide to Mitochondrial Dysfunction" from the Mitochondrial Care Network can be helpful resources for more in-depth information.

4.2 Lifestyle Changes and Dietary Considerations

Dietary modifications and lifestyle adjustments are important aspects of managing mitochondrial dysfunction. Maintaining a balanced diet and leading a healthy lifestyle can help manage symptoms and reduce the progression of mitochondrial illnesses, even if there is no known cure. Here are some important things to think about:

Modifications to Lifestyle

1. Regular Exercise: Exercise on a regular basis can lower the risk of problems and enhance mitochondrial function. To find the right amount of exercise for each person, it's crucial to avoid overdoing it and speak with a healthcare provider.

2. Stress Management: Stress control is essential for maintaining general health, which includes mitochondrial health. Relaxation and stress reduction can be achieved by practices like yoga, deep breathing, and meditation.

3. Adequate Sleep: Getting enough sleep is crucial for preserving the health of your mitochondria and your general wellbeing. Improving the quality of your sleep can be achieved by developing a calming nighttime ritual and a regular sleep regimen.

4. Healthy Diet: Eating a well-balanced diet high in whole grains, fruits, vegetables, lean meats, and

healthy fats can promote general and mitochondrial health. It is imperative to steer clear of processed diets and give fresh, nutrient-dense ingredients top priority.

Dietary Points to Remember

1. Vitamins and Minerals: Coenzyme Q10, vitamin A, vitamin C, vitamin E, and other particular vitamins and minerals may be beneficial for patients with mitochondria. To guarantee safety and proper dosage, it is imperative to speak with a healthcare provider prior to beginning any supplementation.

2. Antioxidants: Antioxidants, like vitamins A, C, and E, can aid in preventing oxidative stress on mitochondrial function. Nuts, fruits, and vegetables can be great sources of these vitamins because they are high in antioxidants.

3. Omega-3 Fatty Acids: Rich in nuts, seeds, and seafood, omega-3 fatty acids can promote mitochondrial health and lessen inflammation.

4. Fiber: Eating a diet high in fiber can promote general health and help keep a healthy gut

microbiome. Good sources of fiber include whole grains, fruits, and vegetables.

It's important to keep in mind that dietary recommendations and lifestyle adjustments might have varying effects on different people. As such, people should consult their healthcare professional before making any major dietary or lifestyle changes. The knowledge and management of mitochondrial illnesses are being advanced by ongoing research.

4.3 Complementary and Alternative Therapies

Despite the paucity of evidence supporting their efficacy, people with mitochondrial dysfunction frequently employ complementary and alternative therapies. The two most popular supplementary and alternative therapies are over-the-counter medications like dietary supplements and homeopathy and self-help methods like yoga and Reiki. It's crucial to remember that these therapies should be utilized in addition to conventional medical care and are not a replacement for it.

Although there isn't enough proof to say that complementary and alternative therapies can stop mitochondrial disease in its tracks, some specialists have noted notable clinical improvements from them. Although the clinical capacity to anticipate therapeutic responsiveness, achieve appropriate medication doses, and quantify benefits in individual patients remains limited, these therapies are generally safe and may relieve certain clinical symptoms.

Before beginning any kind of treatment, it is imperative to talk with a healthcare provider about the use of complementary and alternative therapies. Certain treatments might have possible negative effects or interact with medications. These treatments can also be very expensive, and insurance coverage might not be available.

In conclusion, patients with mitochondrial dysfunction may employ complementary and alternative therapies, although there is insufficient data to determine whether they are beneficial. Patients should utilize these therapies in addition to conventional medical therapy and talk about their use with their healthcare professional. To improve our knowledge of and ability to treat mitochondrial illnesses, research is still being done.

Chapter 5

Living with Mitochondrial Dysfunction

Because mitochondrial dysfunction is a complex condition, living with it can present a number of obstacles. Muscle weakness, exhaustion, heart problems, problems with vision and hearing, and other systemic disorders are only a few of the symptoms that can result from mitochondrial illnesses, which disrupt the synthesis of cellular energy in organs with high energy demands. The main goals of treatment for mitochondrial diseases are to reduce symptoms and delay the course of the illness.

Patients' emotional, psychosocial, and economic well-being can be significantly impacted by mitochondrial illness, which frequently necessitates multidisciplinary care. Because of the heavy weight of the diagnosis, more assistance and care coordination are required. Although there are medications, vitamins, and nutritional supplements available to help reduce symptoms and halt the disease's progression, these interventions vary widely in their efficacy.

To effectively manage their disease, people with mitochondrial dysfunction must collaborate closely with a healthcare team. Regular doctor appointments, hospital stays, and the requirement for social work support to identify and schedule the required resources and assistance may all be part of this. Furthermore, continuing research is essential to improving patient care and learning more about mitochondrial diseases.

In conclusion, receiving care for mitochondrial dysfunction necessitates a multifaceted strategy that includes social, emotional, and medical assistance. Although there are therapies and supporting measures available, their efficacy varies; therefore, further research is necessary to improve patient outcomes and care.

5.1 Coping Strategies for Daily Challenges

It can be difficult to deal with mitochondrial dysfunction on a daily basis, both mentally and physically. Although there are no proven treatments for mitochondrial disorders, there are a number of methods that can help people manage their illnesses and enhance their quality of life. Among these tactics are:

1. Seeking Support: Making connections with patient communities, counseling services, and support groups can offer helpful emotional support and useful guidance for managing the effects of mitochondrial dysfunction.

2. Managing Symptoms: It's critical to collaborate closely with medical professionals to handle certain symptoms, including weariness, muscle weakness, and other systemic issues. A mix of prescription drugs, lifestyle modifications, and rehabilitative therapy may be used to achieve this.

3. Balanced Nutrition: Maintaining general health and energy levels can be facilitated by eating a balanced diet and consulting a nutritionist for specific dietary concerns.

4. Conserving Energy: To manage exhaustion and save energy, people with mitochondrial dysfunction may find it helpful to pace activities, prioritize tasks, and include rest periods.

5. Regular Exercise: Following medical professionals' recommendations to partake in low-impact physical activities will help preserve general health and muscle function.

6. Advocating for Care: People with mitochondrial dysfunction might feel more empowered if they take

an active role in advocating for their own care and keep up to date on the most recent findings and available treatments.

Since the effects of mitochondrial illnesses can differ greatly from person to person, it's critical to address coping tactics individually. By incorporating these tactics into their everyday lives, people can strive to cope with the difficulties brought on by mitochondrial dysfunction while also keeping an optimistic mindset. Hope for the treatment of mitochondrial illnesses in the future is also offered by ongoing research and newly developed therapies.

5.2 Balancing Physical and Mental Well-being

In order to maintain optimal physical and mental health, people with mitochondrial dysfunction must strike a balance. Although there is no treatment for these intricate hereditary illnesses, there are a number of methods that can help control symptoms and enhance quality of life. Here are some important things to think about:

Physical Health

1. Regular Exercise: Exercise on a regular basis can lower the risk of problems and enhance mitochondrial function. To find the right amount of exercise for each person, it's crucial to avoid overdoing it and speak with a healthcare provider.

2. Balanced Nutrition: Both general health and mitochondrial health can be supported by eating a diet rich in fruits, vegetables, whole grains, lean meats, and healthy fats.

3. Managing Symptoms: It's critical to collaborate closely with medical professionals to treat certain symptoms, including weariness, muscle weakness, and other systemic issues. A mix of prescription drugs, lifestyle modifications, and rehabilitative therapy may be used to achieve this.

Mental Health

1. Seeking Support: Making connections with patient communities, counseling services, and support groups can offer helpful emotional support and useful guidance for managing the effects of mitochondrial dysfunction.

2. Stress Management: Stress control is essential for maintaining general health, which includes mitochondrial health. Relaxation and stress reduction can be achieved by practices like yoga, deep breathing, and meditation.

3. Behavioral Interventions: Exercise can help manage stress, anxiety, and depression. It's also one of the finest things you can do for your mitochondria.

Since the effects of mitochondrial illnesses can differ greatly from person to person, it's critical to address coping tactics individually. By incorporating these tactics into their everyday lives, people can strive to cope with the difficulties brought on by mitochondrial dysfunction while also keeping an optimistic mindset. Hope for the treatment of mitochondrial illnesses in the future is also offered by ongoing research and newly developed therapies.

5.3 Building a Support System

Creating a network of support is essential for people with mitochondrial dysfunction since it helps ease their burdens and keep them optimistic despite the condition. The following are essential steps in creating a support network:

1. Get in Touch with Support Groups: Participating in internet forums or support groups can offer priceless emotional support and helpful guidance from people going through comparable struggles.

2. Seeking guidance from a mental health expert can assist people in managing the emotional consequences of having mitochondrial dysfunction, including stress, anxiety, and depression.

3. Educate Yourself and Your Family: Acquiring knowledge about mitochondrial illnesses, their signs, and the therapies that are available can empower individuals and aid in the better understanding of the situation by the patient's family.

4. Collaborate with Healthcare Providers: To manage the disease and guarantee proper care, close collaboration with healthcare providers—including experts and care coordinators—is imperative.

5. Remain Updated: Stay informed on new developments in the treatment of mitochondrial

diseases, as these developments may give patients new hope.

People with mitochondrial dysfunction can better manage the difficulties of their condition and keep a positive outlook by developing a strong support network. There is also optimism for the future management of mitochondrial illnesses due to ongoing research and developing therapeutics.

Chapter 6

Research and Innovations

The goal of current research and innovation in the field of mitochondrial disorders is to create efficient treatments and enhance patient care. Although there isn't a permanent treatment for mitochondrial illnesses at this time, there are a number of research initiatives and cutting-edge treatments that hold promise. Among the important ideas from the sources at hand are:

1. Emerging Therapies: In order to address the underlying molecular causes of mitochondrial illnesses, research is investigating novel therapy techniques, such as nucleic acid-based therapies and other cutting-edge tactics.

2. Drug Development: The creation of possible pharmacological treatments for mitochondrial diseases is the subject of ongoing study. But it's important to note that in order to determine these medications' efficacy and safety, thorough clinical trials are required.

3. Patient-Centered Care and Advocacy: To promote drug development and research for mitochondrial illnesses, patient advocacy organizations and

pharmaceutical corporations are collaborating. Research and clinical trial design are greatly influenced by the opinions and experiences of patients.

4. Supportive Care: Although there are currently few specific treatments for mitochondrial illnesses, the majority of care provided to patients aims to manage their symptoms and enhance their quality of life.

5. Hope for the Future: Despite the present treatment constraints, the research and patient communities are optimistic about the possibility of substantial progress in our knowledge of and ability to treat mitochondrial disorders.

It is imperative that patients and their families remain up-to-date on the most recent advancements in research and treatment methodologies. Working together with medical professionals and interacting with patient advocacy organizations can offer important assistance and access to new knowledge and treatments.

6.1 Promising Advances in Mitochondrial Research

New insights and possible treatment options for a range of complex disorders linked to aging, the environment, and genetics have been made possible by recent developments in the field of mitochondrial research. As a result of these developments, our knowledge of the fundamental roles that mitochondria play in immunology, signal transmission, cellular energy, and the pathophysiology of both primary and secondary mitochondrial illnesses, as well as complex diseases involving mitochondrial malfunction, has grown. Numerous diseases have been linked to mitochondrial dysfunction, which is also a major mechanistic foundation, predictive biomarker, and therapeutic target. Studies have also revealed that lifestyle, environment, and heredity can all have an impact on mitochondrial dysfunction, which may manifest before other clinical symptoms. New approaches to the diagnosis, treatment, and prevention of numerous diseases have been made possible by our growing awareness of the role that mitochondrial malfunction plays.

Regarding therapeutic advancements, vitamins, co-factors, and dietary supplements have been the mainstay of traditional therapy for mitochondrial illnesses, with little evidence of efficacy. Nonetheless, novel treatments are being investigated, such as pharmacological therapy and strategies based on nucleic acids. Preclinical assessments of these novel medicines are encouraging, and human trials employing rigorous methodologies are being conducted. Using the growing knowledge of the pathophysiology of mitochondrial illnesses, the field is also working to create treatments that address the underlying molecular mechanisms of these diseases.

Although there aren't many choices for treating mitochondrial illnesses at the moment, there is ongoing interest in creating viable therapeutic substitutes. The basic understanding of mitochondrial biology has advanced significantly, and there is a growing capacity to carry out significant clinical trials to validate novel treatments. The field of mitochondrial disease research and treatment has seen significant changes due to the application of gene therapy for the correction of mitochondrial DNA abnormalities, the establishment of national mitochondrial disease cohorts, and worldwide collaborations.

In conclusion, new discoveries in the field of mitochondrial research have led to a better understanding of the role that mitochondrial malfunction plays in a number of diseases and have created new opportunities for the creation of focused and efficient treatments. Although the area is still developing, there is optimism for the future management of mitochondrial illnesses due to the advancements in our understanding of mitochondrial biology and the creation of novel therapeutics.

6.2 Clinical Trials and Patient Participation

A crucial step in the research process for creating novel cures and treatments for mitochondrial diseases is conducting clinical trials. Clinical trials are carried out in multiple stages with the aim of assessing the safety and effectiveness of novel treatments and therapies in human subjects. The involvement of patients with mitochondrial illnesses is critical to the advancement of the field, as they are vital collaborators in the research and development of new treatments.

Clinical studies for illnesses related to the mitochondria are usually carried out in specialist centers and need close supervision and control. Clinical trial participants may receive access to novel therapies and treatments that are not provided by routine medical care. Nonetheless, there are hazards associated with clinical trial participation, so patients should carefully weigh the advantages and disadvantages before electing to take part.

Potential pharmacological therapies as well as techniques based on nucleic acids are being investigated as emerging therapies for mitochondrial diseases. Preclinical assessments of these novel medicines are encouraging, and human trials employing rigorous methodologies are being conducted. Using the growing knowledge of the pathophysiology of mitochondrial illnesses, the field is also working to create treatments that address the underlying molecular mechanisms of these diseases.

Pharmaceutical companies and patient advocacy groups are collaborating to progress medicine development and research for mitochondrial illnesses. Research and clinical trial design are greatly influenced by the opinions and experiences of patients. Patients can further the field of mitochondrial research and aid in the development of new treatments and therapies by taking part in clinical studies.

In conclusion, clinical trials play a critical role in the development of novel medicines and treatments for illnesses involving the mitochondria. The involvement of patients with mitochondrial illnesses is critical to the advancement of the discipline, as they are vital collaborators in the research and development of new treatments. To further research and treatment development for mitochondrial illnesses, pharmaceutical companies and patient advocacy groups are collaborating to investigate emerging therapeutics.

6.3 The Future Landscape of Mitochondrial Dysfunction Treatments

Prospects for Treating Mitochondrial Dysfunction in the Future

When mitochondria don't perform as well as they should because of another illness or condition, this is known as mitochondrial dysfunction. Chronic and complicated mitochondrial illnesses can alter your lifestyle and impact several organ systems. Although there isn't a cure for mitochondrial diseases, there are therapies that can lessen symptoms or stop the illnesses' progression.

Identification

Because mitochondrial diseases can resemble other neurological and genetic conditions, diagnosing them can be difficult. To identify mitochondrial illnesses, medical professionals may combine clinical examinations, family histories, and genetic testing.

Intervention

The kind and severity of mitochondrial disorders determine the treatment options. Typical therapy alternatives include the following:

Dietary supplements and vitamins can help reduce symptoms and delay the course of the illness avoiding potentially fatal consequences like liver failure and dysfunction handling symptoms such as dysmotility, hypotonia, cramps, vomiting, reflux, constipation, diarrhea, and muscle weakness taking care of coexisting illnesses such as diabetes, liver failure, parathyroid dysfunction, pancreas failure, and heart defects

To find the best treatment plan for your unique circumstances, you must collaborate closely with your healthcare practitioner. Remember that every treatment has potential adverse effects, and your healthcare professional will go over these with you prior to beginning treatment.

Hope for the Future

The field of mitochondrial illnesses is still being studied, and our knowledge of the condition is growing. Guidelines for patient care standards have been established by the Mitochondrial Medicine Society with the intention of offering direction based on a global agreement of seasoned experts in mitochondrial medicine. Furthermore, by bringing patients and researchers together, groups like MitoSHARE: Mitochondrial Disease Registry promote the development of improved diagnoses, therapies, and cures.

In summary, although there is presently no treatment for mitochondrial disorders, the field of therapeutics for mitochondrial dysfunction appears to be expanding in the future. Patients and their families suffering from these chronic and complex disorders have hope thanks to ongoing research and the development of new therapeutic options.

Chapter 7

Inspiring Stories of Hope and Resilience

Heartwarming Tales of Hope and Fortitude

Physically and mentally, living with mitochondrial dysfunction can be difficult. Numerous issues in the areas of the physical, psychological, social, and spiritual realms frequently affect patients and their families. Nonetheless, there are a lot of heartwarming accounts of resiliency and optimism from people and families who have taken on these difficulties head-on.

A case in point is the narrative of the Mito family, who established the My Mito Mission website to document their experience with mitochondrial illness and offer assistance to other members of the community dealing with the same condition. On their website, patients and their families can find resources, personal experiences, and details about mitochondrial disease.

The Mitochondrial Care Network (MCN), an alliance of medical professionals and patient activists dedicated to enhancing treatment for individuals with mitochondrial disease, is another heartwarming tale. In addition to advocating for improved access to care and therapies, the MCN offers resources for families and patients, such as a recently updated patient handbook.

In spite of their illness, patients with mitochondrial disease also exhibit remarkable fortitude. Even with these obstacles, a lot of patients manage to have happy lives and follow their passions. For instance, despite also having mitochondrial illness, Olympic athlete Chris Nikic made history by being the first person with Down syndrome to finish an Ironman triathlon.

In conclusion, even though having mitochondrial malfunction might be challenging, there are a lot of heartwarming tales of resiliency and optimism shared by people with mitochondrial diseases and their families. These tales serve as a reminder that people with mitochondrial illness can still lead happy lives and achieve their goals if they have the appropriate assistance and tools.

7.1 Patient Success Stories

Testimonials of Successful Patients

Although controlling mitochondrial dysfunction might be difficult, there are numerous encouraging tales of people who have succeeded in doing so.

Devin's tale, in which he was diagnosed with mitochondrial illness as a teenager, is one example of this. Devin has overcome her obstacles to become a support ambassador for the community of people with mitochondrial diseases and has connected with groups like the United Mitochondrial Disease Foundation (UMDF) to feel supported and part of a larger family. Additionally, she has had success controlling her disease by combining prescription drugs, dietary supplements, and lifestyle modifications.

The Mito family is the subject of another motivational tale. They established the My Mito Mission website to document their experience with mitochondrial illness and offer support to other members of the community. On their website, patients and their families can find resources, personal experiences, and details about mitochondrial disease.

A new patient guide is among the services offered to patients and families by the Mitochondrial Care Network (MCN). The MCN is a coalition of medical professionals and patient advocates dedicated to enhancing the quality of care for those with mitochondrial illness.

In conclusion, despite the difficulties associated with having mitochondrial malfunction, there are several patient success stories that give encouragement and hope. Patients who have been successful in controlling their illness frequently attribute their progress to a mix of prescription drugs, dietary supplements, lifestyle modifications, and assistance from groups such as the UMDF and MCN. These tales serve as a reminder that people with mitochondrial illness can still lead happy lives and accomplish their goals if they have the proper assistance and tools.

7.2 Overcoming Challenges: Real-Life Experiences

Numerous obstacles must be overcome when dealing with mitochondrial dysfunction, and personal accounts from people who have gone through these struggles before can provide insightful information and motivation. Patients with mitochondrial illness frequently experience financial, emotional, and psychosocial difficulties, necessitating care coordination and supplementary support. A variety of issues in the physical, psychological, social, and spiritual domains are revealed from the patient's point of view, including coping mechanisms, a sense of loss, and a lack of healthcare. In spite of these obstacles, the community of people with mitochondrial diseases has many heartwarming tales of resiliency and optimism.

Devin, for example, who was diagnosed with mitochondrial disease when he was a teenager, has managed his condition and gone on to serve as an advocate for the mitochondrial disease community. Furthermore, families that have shared their experience with mitochondrial disease, like the Mito family, have helped others going through similar struggles by offering information and support. These accounts demonstrate the tenacity and resolve of people with mitochondrial dysfunction and their families.

In conclusion, the personal accounts of people and families affected by mitochondrial malfunction shed insight on the major obstacles they encounter, such as the financial, social, and emotional costs. These tales, however, also show the population affected by mitochondrial diseases' tenacity and strength, giving others going through comparable struggles encouragement and hope. Patients and families help to increase understanding of the effects of mitochondrial malfunction and offer support to others facing comparable difficulties by sharing their experiences and coping mechanisms.

Chapter 8

Advocacy and Community Engagement

Supporting patients and families impacted by mitochondrial dysfunction involves advocacy and community involvement. Patient advocacy organizations that serve individuals with uncommon genetic illnesses and their families include the North American Mitochondrial Disease Consortium. In order to assess resource and support planning and to provide additional support and care coordination, social work consultants are advised to follow the patient care criteria for primary mitochondrial disease that have been developed by the Mitochondrial Medicine Society. Through the UMDF's mitoSHARE registry, patients can submit their experiences and perspectives about their mitochondrial diseases, which can aid in drug research initiatives and physician education. In general, patients and families impacted by mitochondrial dysfunction need to be supported, and this requires advocacy and community involvement.

8.1 Joining Patient Advocacy Groups

Individuals and families impacted by mitochondrial dysfunction may find great support and knowledge by joining patient advocacy groups. A range of tools and support services are provided by the United Mitochondrial Disease Foundation (UMDF), such as support groups, online forums, educational events, and a patient concierge that helps match people with local mito families or support ambassadors. Furthermore, in order to enhance the standard of mitochondrial patient care and put best practices into effect, mitochondrial physicians and patient advocacy groups have partnered to form the Mitochondrial Care Network (MCN). Patients' advocacy groups oversee and direct the network, which evaluates current gaps in mitochondrial clinical care. By becoming a member of these advocacy groups, people may remain up-to-date on the most recent advancements in the field of mitochondrial dysfunction, connect with others suffering similar issues, and obtain invaluable support.

8.2 Raising Awareness about Mitochondrial Dysfunction

Increasing knowledge of mitochondrial dysfunction is essential to enhancing patient outcomes, diagnosis, and treatment. Informing medical professionals, loved ones, and acquaintances about mitochondrial illness is one way to spread awareness. Receiving a proper diagnosis and treatment might be challenging for patients due to the medical community's lack of knowledge about mitochondrial disease. Additionally striving to increase awareness and enhance the standard of mitochondrial patient care are patient advocacy organizations like the United Mitochondrial Disease Foundation (UMDF) and the Mitochondrial Care Network (MCN). The MCN is a partnership of patient advocacy organizations and mitochondrial doctors with the goal of advancing best practices and raising the standard of care for mitochondrial patients. By becoming a member of these advocacy groups, people may remain up-to-date on the most recent advancements in the field of mitochondrial dysfunction, connect with others suffering similar issues, and obtain invaluable support. Moreover, funding mitochondrial research can increase awareness and result in improvements in diagnosis and therapy.

All age groups are affected by mitochondrial disease, which can result in a variety of life-threatening symptoms such as excessive exhaustion, seizures, and strokes. Lack of funding has made the condition difficult to treat and sluggish to identify, despite its seriousness.

8.3 Participating in Community Initiatives

Engaging in community-based endeavors is vital to promoting consciousness regarding mitochondrial dysfunction and furnishing assistance to individuals impacted by this illness. Here are a few methods for becoming involved in neighborhood projects:

1. Support Groups: To meet people going through similar struggles and exchange experiences, sign up for local or online support groups run by patient advocacy organizations like MitoAction or the United Mitochondrial Disease Foundation (UMDF).

2. Educational Events: Learn about the most recent advancements in mitochondrial dysfunction and treatment by attending conferences, workshops, and educational events hosted by patient advocacy organizations or medical facilities.

3. Fundraising and Awareness Campaigns: Take part in campaigns and fundraising events arranged by local communities or patient advocacy groups to generate money for support services and research.

4. Patient Advocacy Networks: Assist patients by becoming a member of networks like the Mitochondrial Care Network (MCN), a partnership of patient advocacy organizations and mitochondrial doctors that aims to enhance the standard of care for patients with mitochondria and put best practices into effect.

5. Social Media and Online Communities: Participate in online forums and social media groups devoted to mitochondrial dysfunction in order to network, exchange stories, and increase awareness.

6. Local activities and initiatives: Take part in neighborhood, government, or healthcare-related activities and initiatives to promote treatment and research efforts for mitochondrial dysfunction and to increase public awareness of the condition.

By taking part in community activities, people may
help spread the word about mitochondrial
dysfunction, foster the development of support
networks, and enhance the lives of those who are
impacted by the illness.

Conclusion

Embracing Hope and Moving Forward

In conclusion, mitochondrial dysfunction is a difficult and complicated illness that can have a big influence on the lives of those who have it. But there is promise for better diagnosis, care, and patient outcomes because of recent advancements in research and treatment. Patient advocacy organizations are striving to increase awareness, offer support, and enhance the standard of care for patients with mitochondria, such as the United Mitochondrial Disease Foundation (UMDF) and the Mitochondrial Care Network (MCN). People can support these efforts and enhance the lives of people impacted by mitochondrial dysfunction by getting involved in community projects. Even though there is still a lot to learn about mitochondrial dysfunction, people and families impacted by the disorder can overcome obstacles and find a way forward by holding onto hope and using a patient-centered approach.

- **The Power of a Positive Mindset**

People with mitochondrial malfunction and their families can greatly benefit from adopting an optimistic outlook. Even though this illness can be difficult to manage, there is promise for better diagnosis, treatment, and patient outcomes because of recent advancements in research and care. Patient advocacy organizations are striving to increase awareness, offer support, and enhance the standard of care for patients with mitochondria, such as the United Mitochondrial Disease Foundation (UMDF) and the Mitochondrial Care Network (MCN). Through involvement in community projects and interacting with others going through comparable struggles, people can discover a feeling of acceptance and assistance. Keeping an optimistic outlook can also assist people in overcoming obstacles and charting a course for a brighter future. Even though mitochondrial dysfunction can be a complicated and challenging illness, those who are afflicted by it and their families can discover the fortitude and resiliency they need to face the future with confidence by accepting hope and proceeding in a patient-centered manner.

- ## **Looking Towards the Future with Optimism**

Hope is available for those suffering from mitochondrial dysfunction and their families because of recent developments in research and treatment. Patient advocacy organizations are striving to increase awareness, offer support, and enhance the standard of care for patients with mitochondria, such as the United Mitochondrial Disease Foundation (UMDF) and the Mitochondrial Care Network (MCN). Keeping an optimistic outlook can also assist people in overcoming obstacles and charting a course for a brighter future. Through involvement in community projects and interacting with others going through comparable struggles, people can discover a feeling of acceptance and assistance. Even though mitochondrial dysfunction can be a complicated and challenging illness, those who are afflicted by it and their families can discover the fortitude and resiliency they need to face the future with confidence by adopting an optimistic outlook and holding onto hope. For people impacted by mitochondrial dysfunction, there is hope for better diagnosis, treatment, and patient outcomes with ongoing research and support.

Reference

Chang, M. (2019). Mitochondrial Dysfunction: A Functional Medicine Approach to Diagnosis and Treatment. Amazon Digital Services LLC.

Murphy, M. P., & Hartley, R. C. (2018). Mitochondria as a therapeutic target for common pathologies. Nature Reviews Drug Discovery, 17(12), 865-886.

Neuzil, J., Dong, L. F., Rohlena, J., Truksa, J., Ralph, S. J., & Scheffler, I. E. (2013). Mitochondria: the hub of cellular metabolism. Mitochondrial Diseases: Hope for the Future, 1-22.

Parikh, S., Goldstein, A., Koenig, M. K., Scaglia, F., Enns, G. M., Saneto, R., ... & DiMauro, S. (2015). Diagnosis and management of mitochondrial disease: a consensus statement from the Mitochondrial Medicine Society. Genetics in Medicine, 17(9), 689-701.

Schillings, M. L., Kalkman, J. S., Janssen, H. M., van Engelen, B. G., Bleijenberg, G., & Zwarts, M. J. (2007). Experienced and physiological fatigue in neuromuscular disorders. Clinical Neurophysiology, 118(2), 292-300.